Does Back Pain Go Away? 10 Answers To The Most Acute Back Pain Issues

Dr. Robertino Bedenian

Published by Dr. Robertino Bedenian, 2024.

While every precaution has been taken in the preparation of this book, the publisher assumes no responsibility for errors or omissions, or for damages resulting from the use of the information contained herein.

DOES BACK PAIN GO AWAY? 10 ANSWERS TO THE MOST ACUTE BACK PAIN ISSUES

First edition. January 13, 2024.

ISBN: 979-8224699384

Written by Dr. Robertino Bedenian.

Also by Dr. Robertino Bedenian

Fitness Over 60 For Women – How to Stay Fit And Healthy As You Age
Does Back Pain Go Away? 10 Answers To The Most Acute Back Pain Issues
Massage Bible - A Beginners Guide To Western And Eastern Massage Therapy
Going Vegan - How To Vegan Without Going Crazy
Chiropraktik - Was Steckt Eigentlich Dahinter?
Massagen: Ein Überblick Über Westliche Und Östliche Massagetechniken
Natuerlich Abnehmen, Schlank Und Endlich Fit Sein
P.S. Ich Liebe Dich: Wenn Liebe So Einfach Wäre
Was Tun Bei Rückenschmerzen, Bandscheibenvorfall Und Ischiasschmerzen: 10 Antworten Zu Den Häufigsten Fragen Bei Rückenschmerzen
Was Tun Gegen Schlafapnoe, Schlafstörungen Und Schnarchen
Self-Help Books for Women – How to Overcome Depression, Anxiety, Divorce, Addiction, and Trauma
Your Super Gut Feeling Restored – How to Restore Your Life Energy and Overall Health from The Inside Out

DOES BACK PAIN GO AWAY?

10 Answers to The Most Acute Back Pain Issues

Dr. Robertino Bedenian

Download Your FREE Gift Now

Discover 10 Ways to <u>INSTANTLY</u> Relieve Arthritis Pain + 5 New and Natural Ways to Help Your Aches!

As a way of saying "thank you" for your purchase, I'm going to share with you a **FREE Gift** that is exclusive to readers of "Does Back Pain Go Away?"

It will help you instantly and naturally become and stay pain-free!

<u>Click Here to Check it Out</u>[1]

Or

Go Here:

<u>https://arthritispaingone.net</u>

---

1. https://arthritispaingone.net/

ARTHRITIS PAIN
GONE

10 Ways to Instantly Relieve Arthritis Pain

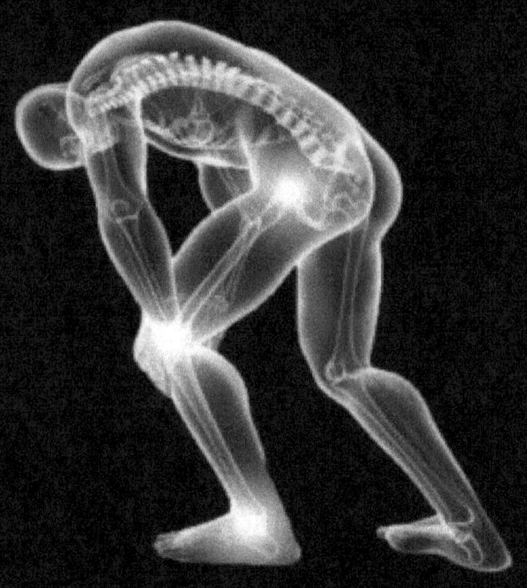

Dr. Robertino Bedenian

CHAPTER 1: WHAT ARE THE CAUSES OF BACK PAIN?

CHAPTER 2: IS BACK PAIN A SERIOUS ISSUE?

CHAPTER 3: HOW TO REDUCE BACK PAIN IN YOUR DAILY JOB

CHAPTER 4: HOW TO AVOID BACK PAIN WHEN RUNNING

CHAPTER 5: WHAT ARE THE BEST METHODS TO RELIEVE BACK PAIN?

CHAPTER 6: WHAT TO DO ABOUT BACK PAIN CAUSED BY STRESS

CHAPTER 7: HOW DO YOU TELL THE DIFFERENCE BETWEEN BACK PAIN AND KIDNEY INFECTION PAIN?

CHAPTER 8: HOW MUCH BACK PAIN IS NORMAL AFTER PREGNANCY BEFORE GETTING CONCERNED?

CHAPTER 9: HOW IS SCIATICA PAIN DIFFERENT FROM BACK PAIN?

CHAPTER 10: WHAT IS THE BEST BED FOR BACK PAIN RELIEF?

THANK YOU!

First, I want to thank you for purchasing this e-book. My sincere desire is that this e-book makes a huge difference in preventing, relieving, and even removing back pain for good. The purpose of this e-book is to give solid answers to the most urgent and acute back pain issues. Due to my intensive research, I found out there are several issues that are addressed time and again when it comes to dealing with enduring back pain. Against this background, I collected the most discussed and contentious questions concerning back pain. As a result, you will find in this e-book the answers to these questions.

CHAPTER 1: WHAT ARE THE CAUSES OF BACK PAIN?

Without the shadow of a doubt, back pain has become one of the most widespread medical issues in the world, and it is second to sick headaches. Most people have suffered back pains. It is usually caused by straightforward tensions and plenty of people need to be cured of this physical suffering. A smooth intensification of muscles that support the backbone and some exercise of the back, along with correct posture with the use of correct lifting secrets and learning the physical limits of the backside could be a big help to end back suffering. Often back pain is due to several diseases or injuries and almost 80 percent of all people experience at least some type of pain in the back. This pain could be continual, brief, serious, or mild. The causes of back pain are often subject to sports injuries, accidents, and muscle strains. Most frequently, the main cause of back suffering is idiopathic or undetermined. However, there are other causative factors, which worsen the feeling of discomfort. The lower portion of the back is being considered the midpoint of gravity in the human body. It is a fact that it is the lower back that holds the heaviness and stress as compared to the other portions of the body. The pain originates from the muscles that were strained because of incorrect mechanics of the body and body movements that are awkward. Unfortunately, for most of us back pain exercises often contribute to producing only short-term relief from back pain. But why are the relieving results only temporary? To understand this, you first need to understand what brings about back pain. As a result, you will develop an understanding of why some exercises are considered to be most effective and why others are of minor benefit. But before we jump into the best exercises in chapter 5 let us take a look at the real reasons for back pain. There are only three causes that trigger back pain. The reason so many people fail to apply the proper pain relief techniques is that they miss out on determining the genuine reason for their pain. Most people assume that backache is due to a tight musculature. This is one reason, but just one. If your body has tight muscle tissues, you will likely possess muscles with much less strength, too. However, the way your blood and your nerve impulses are distributed to the muscles is critical. So, it is not only about physical power. This combination of both weakened as well as tightened muscle groups are known as muscle imbalance. Remember, three main things that cause back pain, with muscle imbalance being one of them. So, what are the other two reasons? The two other sources of back pain are joint imbalances and trigger points. Whenever joints are hindered to move freely or are restricted in their natural movement, these are known as joint imbalances. Moreover, they can even induce actual muscle imbalance, too. As a consequence of joint imbalance, muscle groups need to work harder to meet their daily challenges. As a result, they become tense resulting in a painful condition. If this condition is kept up for a long period, muscle tissues will finally be worn out. In this case, injuries will be unavoidable, and then trigger points will build up. These little nodules of muscle spasm can easily send pain out of the backbone and to the muscle. So, these three factors (muscle imbalance, joint imbalance, and trigger points) and especially the combination of those since each one can certainly produce the other, are the main reasons for back pain. It will not be sufficient to battle one factor. To experience final back pain relief, you will need to eliminate all three issues. In chapter 5, we are going to discuss the best exercises to achieve those long-term results for back pain relief. Depending on the duration back pain can be categorized as follows: chronic, acute, and sub-acute. As a rule, acute pain is generally due to minor injuries, lasts a maximum of four weeks, and may lead to sub-acute pain - lasting as much as twelve weeks. In case your pain should last more than twelve weeks, you need to consult a doctor since the causes could be more complex. Should you experience low-back pain after sitting for an extended time, sharp pain in the neck, stiffness along the spine, aching, or when the pain radiates from the back down the legs or buttocks, you probably need to consult your physician regularly, i.e. you should consider scheduling an appointment together with your physician. If back pain is closely followed by other symptoms, then back pain must not be considered as a temporary inconvenience but is to be treated with higher concern. Symptoms will vary. However, they often include high fever, unexplained or unintended weight reduction, and immunosuppression. For those who have suffered recent trauma, are utilizing intravenous drugs, have osteoporosis, are experiencing a focal neurological deficit, possess a history of cancer, or when the pain has not stopped in six weeks, then consulting your physician immediately is crucial. Experiencing pain in the dorsal region is considered a medical emergency if you are over seventy years of age, or if you have suffered mild trauma, and you are fifty-plus-years old. During a medical visit, you will be asked some questions. Some of them could make you feel uncomfortable in addition to the questions about your pain and about any other possible symptoms you might be experiencing. The doctor's goal is to comprehend your medical history before he can outline your remedy guide. Generally, according to this health background, along with a physical examination, a doctor will be able to establish the reason for your back pain. To determine your physical shape, you will be asked to strength testing on a treadmill, checking reflexes, responses to heat, touches, and pinpricks. Do not be astonished if you need to expose to blood tests, X-rays, MRI or CT scans to verify or establish the precise cause. Any kind of pain is very troubling, especially in the back area, as it could significantly intervene with your abilities to work, exercising, or even standing. However, as there is a proper treatment for each condition, which induces pain in the cervical, thoracic, lumbar, or sacral region of the back, you should not be concerned about it too much. Most typical actions for decreasing pain include painkillers, special physical exercises, anti-inflammatory drugs, and alternative remedies like acupuncture, massage therapy, music treatment, posture courses, spinal cord adjustment, and breathing methods. Most people can cure easily back stiffness with rest, drugs, and some other easy cures at home. But if your back pains in a distressing manner you need to consult your doctor and ask some for medicines or more complete physical care. There are steps in healing back pains. Treat your trouble in the most traditional means. Always bear in mind that surgical operation should only be your last resort. Taking a rest can reduce the discomfort, and skipping this simple step will probably make your pain worse. So, one or two days of complete rest in treating back sufferings from sprains and strains is highly recommended. Treating back pain is not so complicated, but you need to take steps when you face back pain. Treating it lightly could have hazardous effects in the long run. So, make sure you will not experience any additional complications by taking these symptoms seriously. If you do so, there will be a good chance that your back pain is relieved or even removed entirely.

CHAPTER 2:
IS BACK PAIN A SERIOUS ISSUE?

Let us assume that you had back pains for years, should you still really be worrying about it? After all, as mentioned above more than eighty percent of individuals suffer from back pain someday in their life. Therefore, while you grow older back pain occurs more often, and it is more often than not persistent. Therefore, if it is very widespread, is it worth distressing about it? Should we merely agree to it and realize that our lifetimes will probably be filled with agony as we grow older? You breathe in and out, and it is also sore. Every time the heart beats you feel pain. Thinking it is a crippling process, you can even feel your kidneys, liver, intestinal tract, stomach racked with pain each time this function. So, why might back pain end up being any different? Indeed, it is right that normal operating processes ought to be pain-free. If you felt uncomfortable anytime your own heart had a beat, you would be not simply concerned but completely anxiety stricken. There should be no difference when it comes to back pain. You should not suffer from any pain anywhere else. Pain is not natural and part of your body's function order. Quite the contrary, it always signals that there is something wrong. Something in your body is out of balance. Each physical activity you decide to do should be completely pain and ache-free, from the time you get up until you hit the sack and wake up once again. Normality is different from being common. So, back pain might be common for many people, but it is not normal. If this was normal, then you would be supposed to suffer pain each instant through the day while every process in your body did its day-to-day tasks. Back pain should not be present. It should be an issue you cannot afford to underestimate. That is why you need to take appropriate steps now before it becomes a chronic disease, which is not curable anymore. Just because other people are battling with back pain does not suggest you also need to run this race. Apply simple procedures, which you can use at home, that can help balance your muscles and joints. Back pain relief is a straightforward action that takes minimal energy. All investments take some time, funds, or work. So, back pain relief is not different. However, this investment of time and energy will pay out tremendously. You get enormous rewards by simply spending a small amount of effort and time now and the outcomes are for many years. Yet again, a lasting cure is still necessary to get rid of both symptoms as well as the cause. Just minutes every week or two can certainly keep a healthy spine easily. And that is the major goal. There are only three areas you have to focus on. First, you have to make sure that the joints move properly as well as the pelvis is balanced. Second, that muscles, which might be tighter, are stretched properly. And third, you need to encourage the nerve as well as blood circulation to muscular areas that are weak. The final action though is important. You should ensure that your whole body is quite healthy and balanced and that it has the ability to recover. It may well seem complex but these simple steps need very little time and effort. If you pursue these basic guidelines, you will enable to enjoy your elder years free of pain. Consider back pain relief being an investment that is well worth every penny of your time, effort, and hard work. A preferred option for low-back pain relief is exercising regularly. Exercises are one of the most important self-treatments for low-back pain relief. They even guarantee pain relief. Exercises that are specific for your particular low-back pain symptom will usually give you fast relief as they strengthen the core muscles that support the spine, improve the flexibility in the spine, and support posture. Non-impact aerobic exercises also have many benefits. However, the focus should be on safe exercises. If you are unsure, you should always consult a professional back pain adviser. Stretching exercises will also remarkably contribute to your quest for low-back pain relief. Stretching should be carried out slowly, concentrating on the lower back, hips, quadriceps, and hamstrings. Note that stretching exercises will naturally cause pain. In this only case, pain is indeed natural and not common because this pain has to be considered pain from the muscle being stretched. So, stretching triggers a healthy pain process. As a result of this process, pain that is involved due to the stretching exercises is to be considered natural. If you feel pain in any other areas while doing these exercises, you should immediately stop. But if the stretching exercises are done properly, they should increase your flexibility in the region of 20% within the first month and reduce low-back pain considerably.

CHAPTER 3:
HOW TO REDUCE BACK PAIN IN YOUR DAILY JOB

When it comes to preventing back pain in your daily job routine, posture is critical. Posture, or to be exact, improper posture is claimed to be one of the factors that result in back pain, but it is also merely one cause. The way you use to be sitting at work and the way you are standing in line while waiting has a massive impact on your back and spine health. The short-term impact may be insignificant but in the long run, your back will suffer damages. Back pain will gradually increase, as your posture gets more and more slouched. Think about the workplace these days whereby many people now sit slumped over their Laptop for very long hours performing stress-filled work. Pain will build up. It is simply a matter of time. However, if bad posture was the major cause, then every man or woman in your job environment would be predestined to have back pain as a consequence. Simply, because everybody around you is performing the identical workload, is subject to the identical stressful workplace, and is even slouching above the same Laptop. As already mentioned, sometime in your lifetime you have an eighty percent chance of battling back pain, according to statistics. Nevertheless, posture is not the key reason for backache. As a rule, backache is due to three main challenges. When these challenges happen to be existing in your daily life routine, then your posture could aggravate these and permit backache to occur possibly with greater regularity or maybe more significantly. So, what are these factors? We have already mentioned these in chapter one: muscular tension, as well as tissue weakness, are to be counted among these factors that induce back problems. Second, there is joint instability, which prevents the joints from moving readily. And third, trigger points are also spasms of muscle fibers within the muscle itself. Putting together all of these factors enables backache to build up. In addition, having a lousy posture at your workplace or perhaps elsewhere will make pain a lot easier to progress within your body. So, back pain comes along with these imbalances. Against this background, improper posture triggers a rise of pressure on the spine, and you might experience back pain more regularly than before. So, what is the correct answer and what are the simple strategies to reduce back pain in your daily job routine to prevent long-lasting back pain? By now, you might have already tried to keep your posture by simply sitting up straighter while you are pursuing your daily tasks. But unfortunately, you might have caught yourself just a few minutes later with your shoulders hanging forward and your head probably inclining towards your desk. As a result, you start to feel your upper back tensing. The best back pain prevention and relief strategies are simple and do not only work but also do not require a lot of time from your day. You can also take effective steps that can help by simply getting up from your chair and taking a stroll around your office room. Just, this one thing will prevent or diminish your pain. But the key is: you need to take action! You should be willing to enhance your posture by performing basic things just like this. To avoid backache in the long run you need to take it one step further. You will want to eliminate every structural imbalance. Back pain relief does not have to be challenging. Just altering your sitting posture and getting from your chair frequently can and will have a significant impact on your back health. Removing the imbalances that are found in the spine remains the simplest way to generate a permanent improvement in your back pain. In chapter five, we will focus on the best exercises how these imbalances are to be removed most effectively.

CHAPTER 4:
HOW TO AVOID BACK PAIN WHEN RUNNING

Low-back pain is the most common pain syndrome in the United States today. Moreover, it is not only limited to people who pursue sedentary jobs. Even runners and many athletes suffer from this condition regularly. Their suffering is usually due to a combination of physical causes and altered running or walking biomechanics that may be causing the painful condition. The main physical causes of this condition are as follows:

1. Over-pronated or supinated (high arch) feet:

The pronation of the foot is both a natural motion attenuation and a movement towards the inside. In cases of over-pronation, the foot's edge tends to be over-bent exposing the ligaments, tendons, and joints to an overload of pressure. This over-pronation is due to various causes, such as a foot deformity, obesity, or excessive fatigue. Over-pronation happens to occur more with running people who are beginners because their support apparatus is not yet sufficiently trained. With over-pronation, running shoes use to wear out particularly in the medial area (inside of the shoe). Supination, however, occurs much more rarely. With supination, the stress load tends to travel in the opposite direction. In this case, running shoes use to wear out in the lateral area (outside of the shoe). Mostly, this is due to an arched foot. Most running shoe manufacturers offer models with built-in pronation support.

2. Tight hip flexor:

Tight hip flexor muscles cause increased pressure on the lumbar spine. Standing frequently in a hollow back position, you may encounter back problems. For this reason, make sure that the hip is extended regularly to prevent distortion. This exercise should be done to relax the hip flexor muscles:

Go into the one-legged knee level stand and then shift your weight slowly to the front leg. This way, the pelvis is pushed forward and down while your back leg is being stretched at the hip joint. Be sure to tighten the abdominal muscles. Thus, you prevent the pelvis to take a hollow back position. Feel the stretch in the front area of the hip of the back leg. Do the same exercise with the other leg. See the exercise demonstration below:

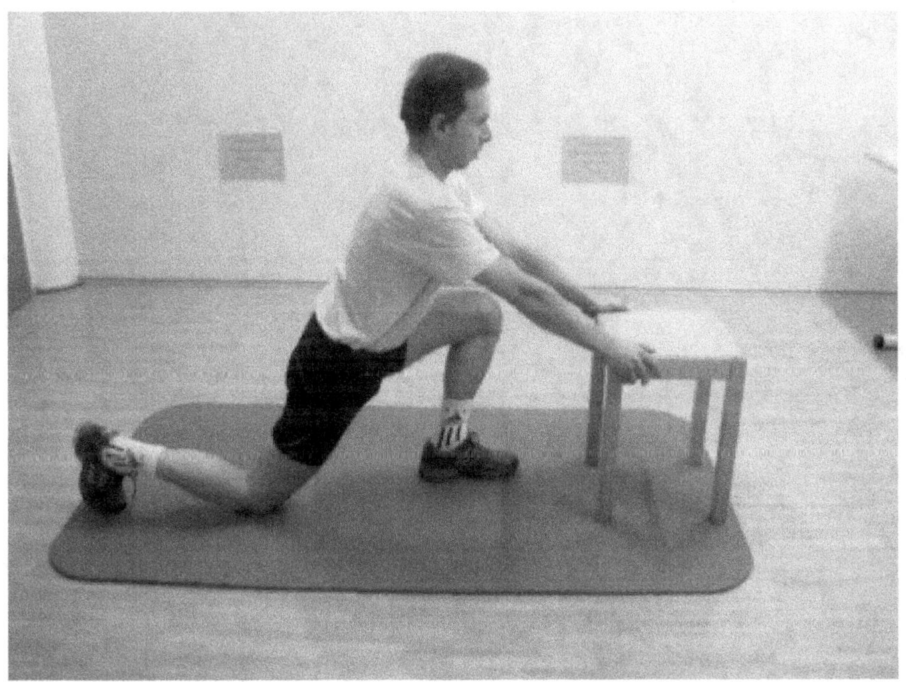

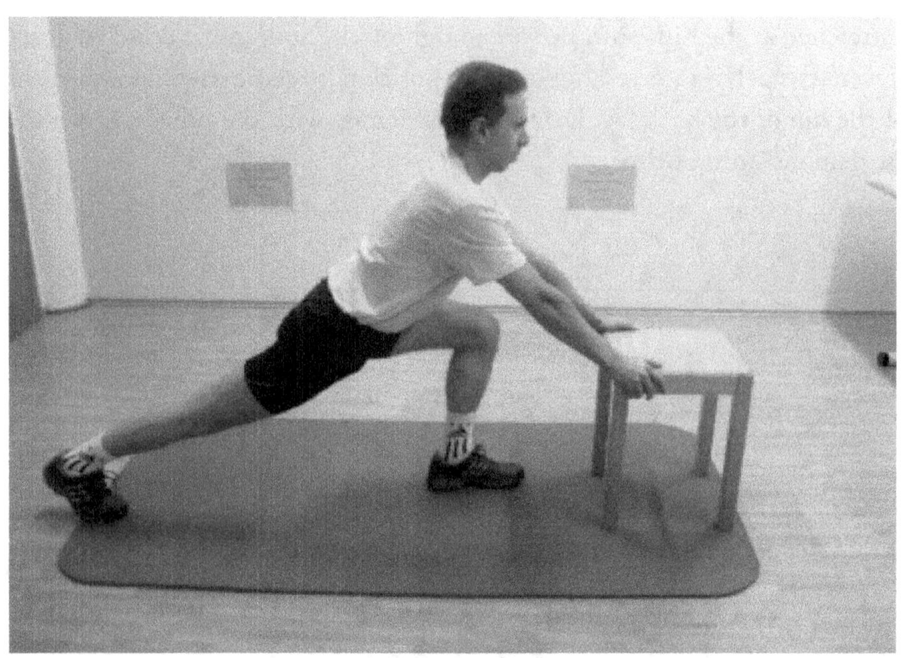

3. Excessively flat or arched lumbar spine:

The lumbar spine is located at the lowest area of the spine. Walking constantly in an upright position puts severe pressure on the lumbar spine. Normally, the lumbar spine is supposed to be only slightly arched. If the arch, however, increases, you will most likely suffer pain. In some cases, the natural arch of the lumbar spine could even vanish completely. As a result, the lumbar spine levels off entirely. This is called a *flat lumbar spine*. Massage and coordinated exercise training as parts of physiotherapy are very promising for back pain relief in the lumbar spine. In addition, a specific muscle- strengthening and muscle-building workout for the spine are highly recommended. Do the following exercise to support your lumbar spine:

Lie flat on your back. Bend your legs at a 90-degree angle and lock your knees. Press with your right hand on your bent knees and push them down toward the right side of your body. Stretch your left arm and press it toward the opposite side while your head is also turned in this direction. Repeat the exercise on the other side. See the exercise demonstration below:

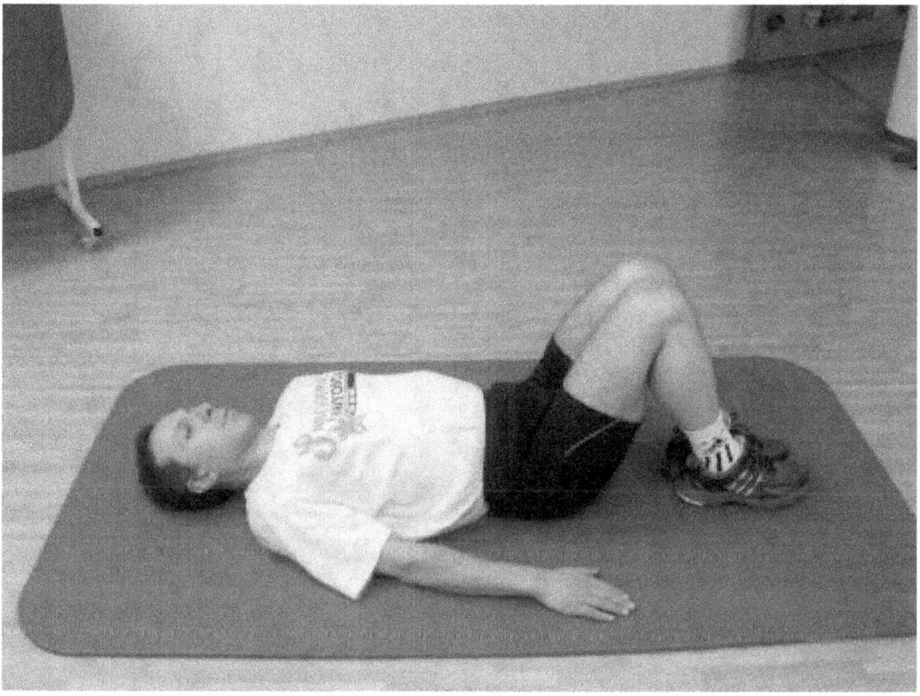

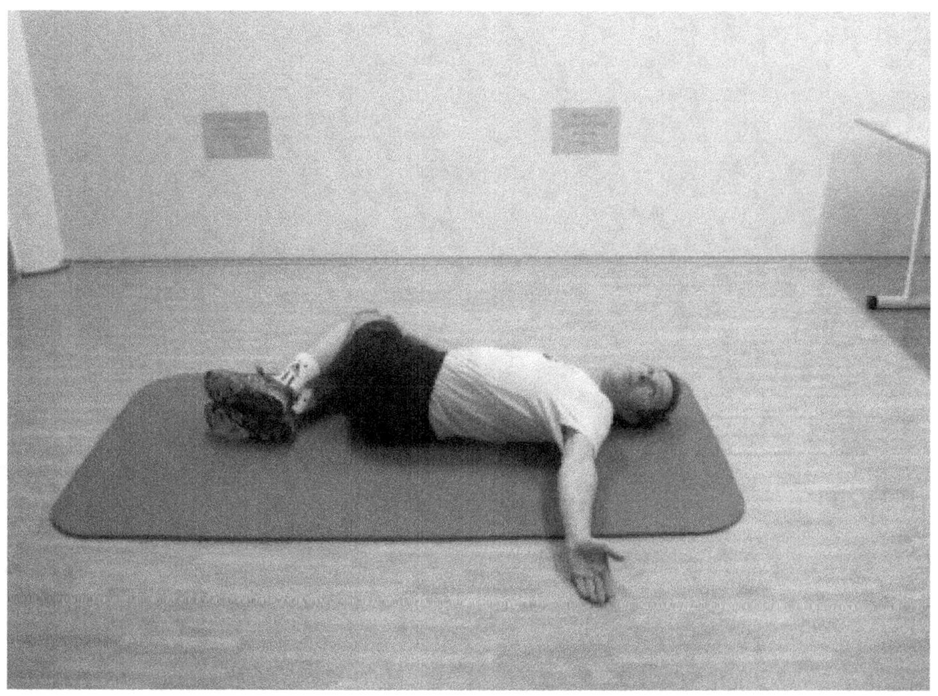

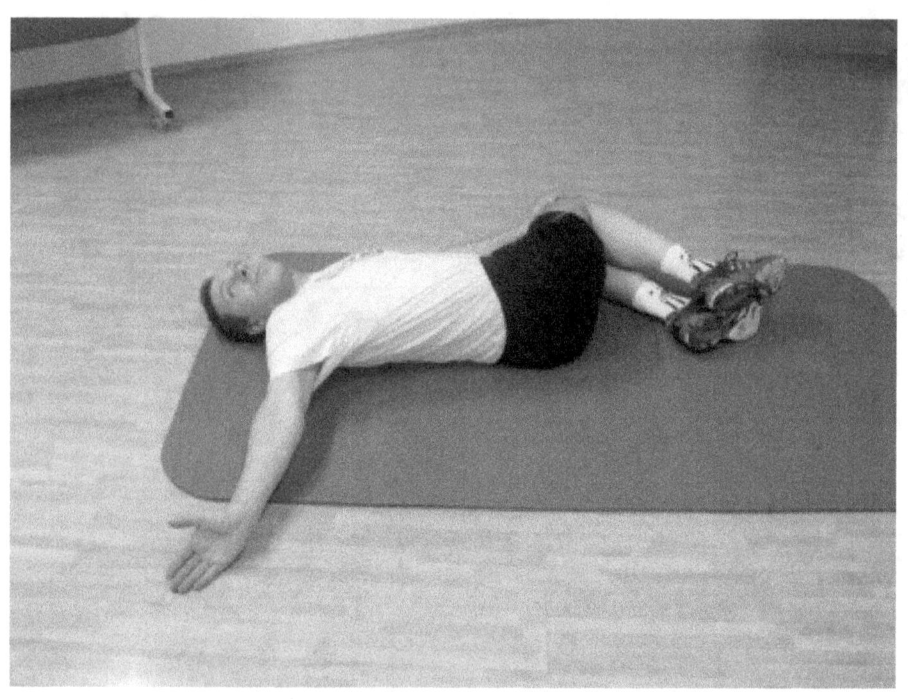

4. Joint restrictions in the thoracic spine:

In comparison to neck and lower-back pain, pain in the thoracic spine and ribs are less likely. Because of their proximity to the heart and lungs, it is difficult to determine the cause of this pain. Suffering from thoracic spine pain may also cause difficulties in breathing, heart stabbing, nausea, and heart palpitations. For this reason, in such cases, it is advisable to consult a heart specialist. If, however, he rules out any heart issues as an explanation for the complaints, the back is to be examined next. Pain in the thoracic spine is usually due to a continuous overload of the surrounding muscle or blockage of the small vertebral joints or joints of the ribs. Such congestion or blockage may result from a poor sleeping position, wrong or hyper-active engagement in sports. The heavy physical workload in a bent posture, excessive workout, or exposure to severe cold may also account for this kind of pain. In such cases, massage and heat treatments with hot roll, mud or paraffin treatment to promote muscle relaxation are highly recommended.

5. Weak glutes:

Shortened and weak glutes account for limited extensions of the hip and thigh muscles accompanied by a restricted range of movement while running. Thus, the steps become smaller, and the body's gravity is not distributed optimally. As a consequence, your knees are exposed to an overload of stress resulting in poor performance and limited mileage. To promote the mobility of the muscles the following exercise is recommended:

Sit upright on the floor and stretch your legs out. Now bend your right and your left leg. Then put your bent left leg on your bent right leg. Now grab the knee of your right leg slowly with both arms and pull it towards your chest. Doing this exercise, you will feel a stretching in the right buttock. Now, do the same exercise with your left knee. See the exercise below:

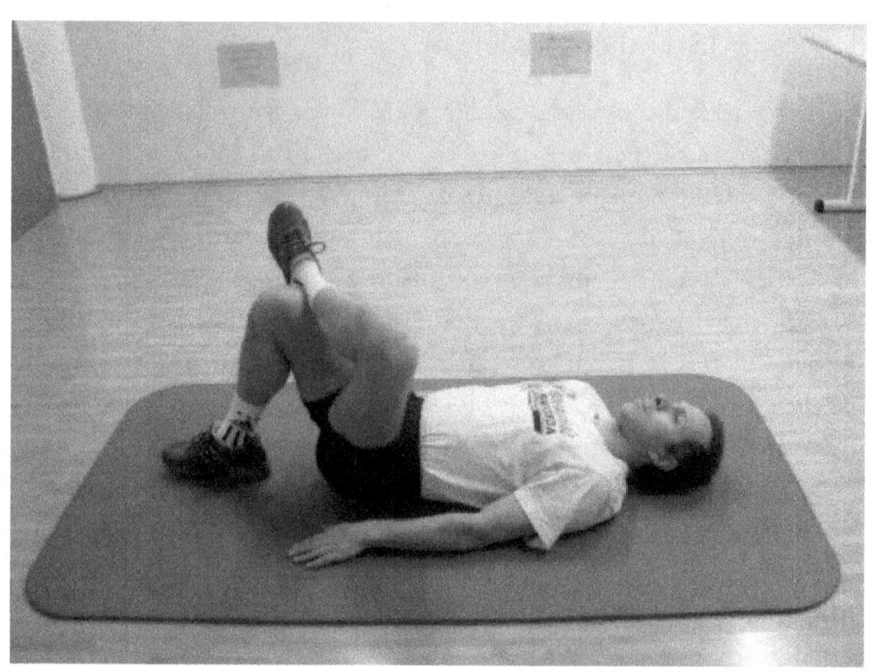

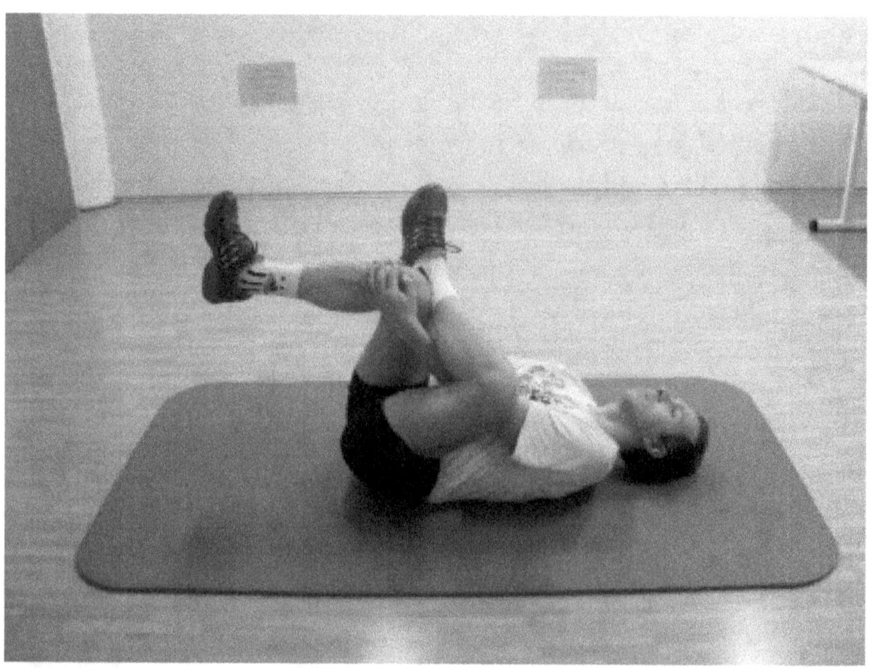

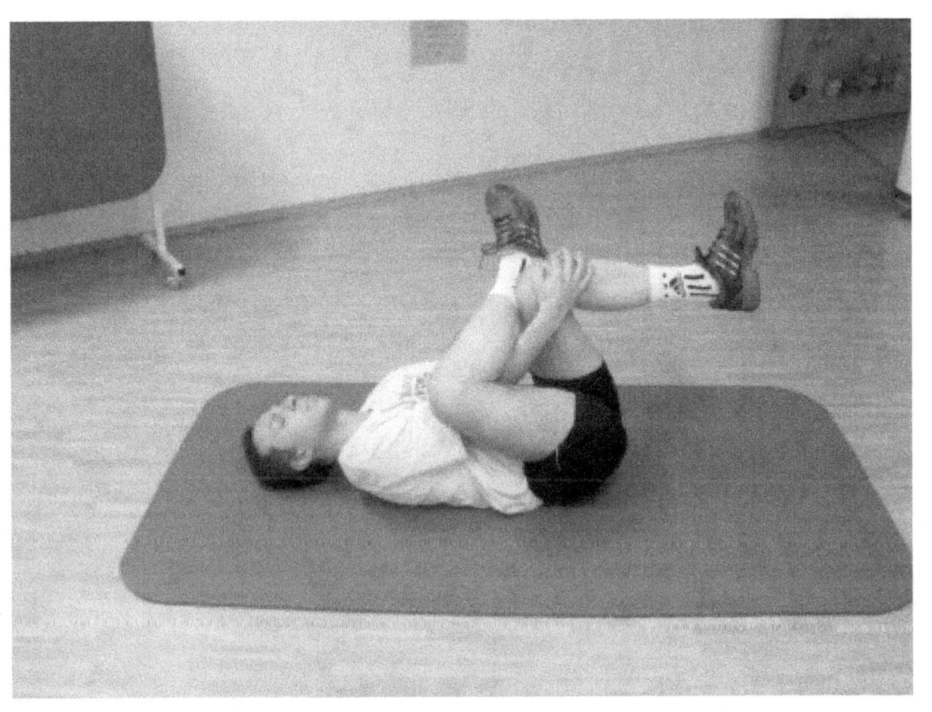

6. Tight hamstrings:

To release tension in the hamstrings, do the following exercise:

First, stand in an upright position. Now bend your right leg and pull it with both hands toward your chest. Then take with both hands your right foot and pull the bent right knee behind your buttocks. Pull in your stomach. Now push your pelvis forward until you feel the stretching in the right thigh muscles. Repeat this exercise with your left leg. See the exercise below:

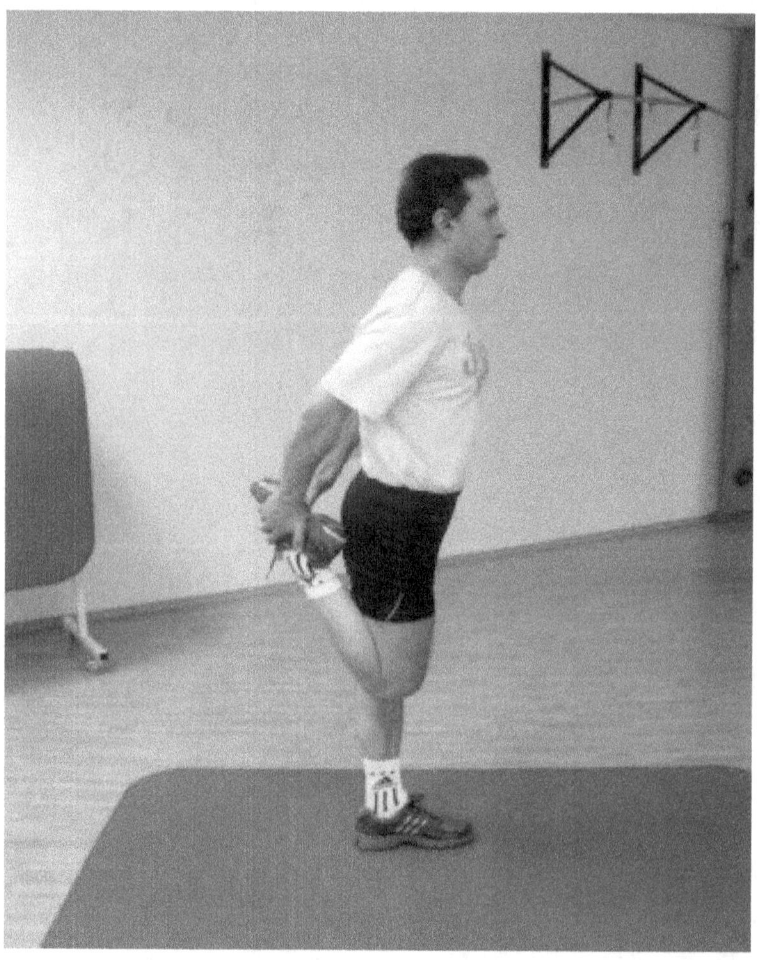

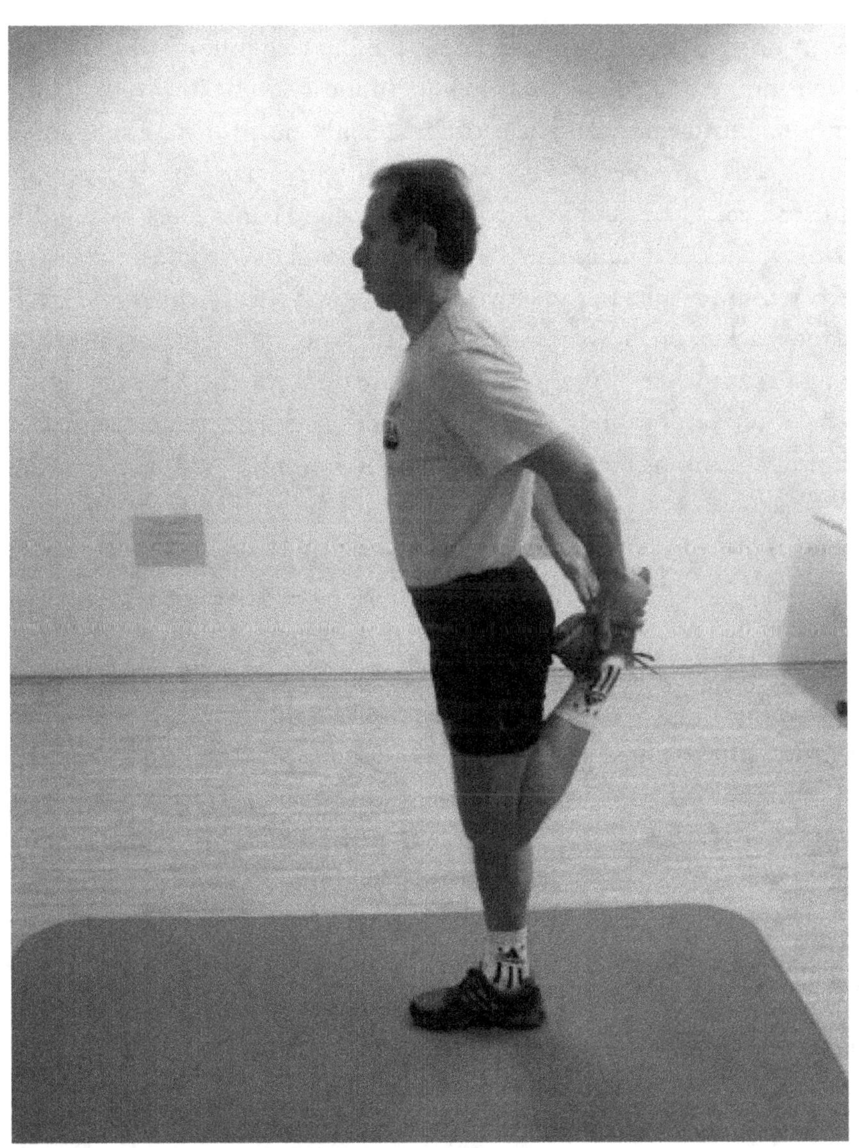

Hip extension firing pattern when extending the hip (leg-pulling through and back) during running or walking the glutes are supposed to be involved in most of the extension. The low back and hamstrings are only meant to have supportive qualities during this movement. With many runners, this pattern is not strictly followed due to weak glutes and overactive low back and hamstrings. When this happens, the low back and hamstrings are exposed to an overload of stress. As a consequence, tension results in these two structures and this is why runners will suffer from low-back pain. However, low-back pain is not only due to a physically poor running performance. Other non-physical reasons for the poor condition could also have a hazardous impact on the runner's back and spine health. For instance, improper running technique, worn-out or improper running shoes, and increasing mileage too fast could result in devastating damages in the long run. If you feel any of the non-physical reasons may be an issue, you definitely should contact your running store or coach to address them. Another huge problem in today's society is sitting too much. Even as active runners, sedentary activities constitute much of our day while at work and home. Research studies show that sitting accounts for 40% of stress on the discs and muscles of our lumbar spine. This is the main cause of chronic low-back pain. From a physical standpoint, the best way to prevent low-back pain is to battle the causes by performing stretches and exercises. That is the only way to handle these dysfunctions. Strengthening for the glute, foot/ankle and core is critical. Ignoring this is just careless. Secondly, you need to check out if you have excessively tight hamstrings, flat or high arches, and unstable ankles. Even altered curves to the lumbar spine (too flat or too arched), tight hip flexors, and other muscular imbalances will expose the lumbar spine to undue stress. Glute strengthening exercises activate the glute max, the main muscle group responsible for glute function and hip extension. Side leg lifts strengthen and activates the glute medius, the main muscle group in providing hip stability during one- leg stance and running. In case you should suffer from low-back pain, conservative treatment usually does a great job of freeing you from your pain. If you are a runner, you should familiarize yourself with the techniques above to keep enjoying running. Now, let us focus on the best methods to relieve back pain.

CHAPTER 5:
WHAT ARE THE BEST METHODS TO RELIEVE BACK PAIN?

Back pain exercises work well supposed that they have been carefully selected to address every trigger. In any case, it is crucial to integrate techniques that target all three factors so you will experience long-term recovery. We have already discussed these three factors in chapter one.

To be straightforward, there is no way to find the only exercise that battles all issues simultaneously. Thus, you should not waste your time hoping that you might discover the unique and particular exercise to be the miracle cure. Because simply there is no one. However, if you realize that to get rid of these issues you have to apply several back pain exercises, you are already on your best way to achieve your goal. As your back pain is the result of a combination of issues, there are also different strategies to be applied as a consequence.

However, you do not need to apply a wide array of exercises. You only need to use the most highly efficient exercises for back pain that are discussed below. These are the ones that cover every cause and not only just one. By using a combination of these exercises, you will be able to achieve a pain and ache-free back sooner than you might think.

One of the most effective strategies to ease the agony of back pain is with stretches for low-back pain. Since most examples of back pain are due to muscle imbalances or slumping posture (which often ends up in muscle imbalances in the long run), stretching will help you to boost under-used muscles and release the strain to tight or contracted muscles.

So, let us take a look at the most highly efficient stretches for low-back pain that you need to pursue:

1.Piriformis Stretch:

So, what is that? Your piriformis is a muscle located deep within your pelvis. If it becomes too tight, it can clamp down on your sciatic nerve. As a consequence, you suffer from agony in your hips or butt sooner or later. The piriformis stretch counteracts this tension that will eventually help to release the piriformis. If you want to watch a demonstration of this exercise, I recommend watching the video of **Dr. Steven Hoffmann** (https://for-ever-fit.net/piriformis-stretch). He is showing how to exercise the piriformis stretch the right way.

2. Cobra Stretch:

As a rule, most of our days we spend sitting, and unfortunately, many of us use to slouch. So, we tend to have an improper posture while we do it. We have already talked about this issue before in chapter three. As a consequence, muscles are automatically trained to pull us forward i.e. evoke us to slouch and cause back pain. So, the Cobra Stretch is meant to pull your muscle in the opposite direction. This yoga exercise can undo some of the bad posture habits while sitting all day. In this case, I recommend watching a short demonstration by **Scott White** (https://for-ever-fit.net/cobra-stretch).

3. Swan Dive:

Whenever the sciatic nerve gets pinched somewhere along its course through the body it will cause back pain. If this happens, the Swan Dive should be exercised. The purpose of this yoga stretch is to essentially tighten the nerve and release it regardless of the sort of kink that it might have got stuck in. **Silver Sport** (https://for-ever-fit.net/swan-dive) presents a short but very helpful video exercising the Swan Dive.

If you pursue these three steps regularly, you will loosen up your sciatic nerve and relieve the agony you are feeling. Of course, it takes a little time to see any results. So, please stick with them for a fortnight when required. You will see results.

Moreover, you should complete your stretching exercises by flexing the muscles, tendons, and ligaments. This should be completed for a minimum of six months in case you should suffer from chronic back discomfort.

Due to physical exercise, the distribution of nutrients inside the spinal column is stimulated as well as the bodily processes are activated. As a consequence, you will experience that your back becomes flexible and robust, making you much less susceptible to recurring back discomfort.

As soon as the muscles are exercised the muscles will start strengthening. Nevertheless, keep in mind that your physique also requires a couple of days of rest, as an excessive amount of exercising may be stressful.

CHAPTER 6:
WHAT TO DO ABOUT BACK PAIN CAUSED BY STRESS

Nowadays, it seems that stress has penetrated every area of life. Family and relationship issues, financial struggle, health concerns, and the increasing challenge we face in our jobs are causing our hormone stress levels to rise in an unprecedented way. The fact that everything in the world is not only subject to change but that things are also changing faster than ever before is causing much more stress today. Unfortunately, we are not able to eschew stress at some point in our lives. However, we need to find ways to diminish the hazardous impact of stress. The good news is that there are a variety of ways at your disposal that help to reduce the impact of stress on the body. If you are looking for a more convenient way to counteract stress symptoms, then you should focus on the benefits of a massage chair. But before you consider this let us take a closer look at what stress is really about.

To many people, the term "stress" is associated with a physically damaging condition. Stress is a quite ordinary reaction of the body to situations that require the body to engage the next gear level. So, stress forces us to leave our comfort zone to proceed in several areas of our lives. It enhances us to become productive, which certainly is to be considered positive. Second, stress is our natural reaction to self-protection. On the one hand, whenever we are exposed to stressful situations, it activates our body to react. This reaction gives our bodies an unambiguous command: "Get ready for action." On the other hand, swamping our body constantly with stressful situations could have a disastrous impact on our health in the long run.

Being stressed can be due to a wide range of things, situations, and circumstances. However, the same situations people face don't necessarily trigger the same stress levels. As people are different so are their reactions to specific situations. For instance, not being able to pay the rent may cause some people to become entirely distressed while other people use to handle this situation for what reason at all with fewer concerns. However, more complex issues like our relationships with others – as everybody needs relationships to exist - could more likely cause us to be exposed to at least more similar stress symptoms. So, whatever the reason may be, our bodies' response to it is stress, yet to a different extent.

So, how does the body react to stress? Most interestingly, there is often a fight or flight reaction to stress. The way the body responds to stress is either by fighting or by fleeing from it. The body's goal is self-protection, and these are the strategies it hopes to succeed with. Whenever the body is about to face imminent danger, he will have these two strategies at hand sending out his command: "Get ready for fighting or fleeing." Today, the situations we face will be less likely to expose us to a physical danger but much more to psychological danger.

So, is it so easy to reprogram our bodies to deal with psychological stress? Our bodies have been accustomed over a long time to react to stress as if there is an imminent bodily danger ahead. However, if the source of stress is psychological, then the approach to stress has to be different, too. Most of the stress we experience is due to the way we think about the problem. Do we consider this situation as temporary, solvable, and manageable? Or do we categorize this problem as permanent, insolvable, and devastating? The answer to this is crucial. The way we think about it determines the way we will feel about it. The way we feel about it accounts for the stress hormone level. So, whenever we face a psychological issue, we will hardly be able to fight or flee from it as if it were a physical problem. As for the psychological issue, we will have to approach differently by taking inventory about the way we think about this situation. If the way we think about it makes us feel miserable, then we will need to make some adjustments in our minds. Our goal is to change the way we FEEL about it. And this starts by changing the way we THINK about it.

However, when you face stressful situations, by even applying this appropriate strategy, you might not experience a sudden relief. So why not? Because it takes some time to reprogram your pattern of thought. But you can and will succeed quicker than you might think. In this situation in which stress is not resolved, the body's reaction to it is a rise of tension.

As tension is to be considered as a conglomerate of energy the way to fight the disastrous effects of stress on the body is by releasing this excess baggage of energy. Exercises and massage therapy work in a tremendous way to get rid of this unhealthy energy.

So, whenever you come under stress, there is only one cure, which is relaxation. Relaxation is the remedy to stress. Massage chairs are a great way to provide relaxation. Massage chairs help you to relax your mind so it does not focus on the cause of stress. Relaxing your mind is the best method to clear your way for reprogramming your mind. Changing your pattern of thought should be your goal. Relaxation is the best possible jump-start to make sure to get there.

As for stress, timing is critical, too. To battle the impact of stress most effectively, you will need to defend yourself from the flying arrows of stress, so to speak, while these arrows are still on their flight path. So, you need to fight stress as soon as you realize that it starts building up. In case you should miss this starting point, you will find it harder to counteract as stress starts to rise to a higher level becoming more powerful with you becoming more susceptible to its damages.

Listening to soothing music is an incredibly effective way to relax. As manufacturers of massage chairs have realized the stress-relieving impact of soothing music you will often find incorporated music players with headphones on massage chairs to enhance the relaxation of the mind. Remember: your thoughts determine the way you feel. Given this, music is a great assistant to distract the mind and thus empty it of its negative thoughts.

Body, mind, and soul are inseparably related to each other. If one of them suffers, the other one will be affected, too, in some way. But the opposite is true as well. Have you ever realized that when your mind is relaxed that your body also relaxes? This is the pivot when it comes to reducing stress. If your mind becomes exhausted by meditating on the same problems time and again, then it will be difficult to relieve the tension in the body. As a consequence, the muscles maintain their stiffness and thus become very resistant to the penetration of massage therapy.

As already mentioned above, stress is unavoidable. The question is how you counteract the effects of stress. Massage chairs help to provide a natural way to release the tension of negative stress. They also support you in reducing tension in the body before your stress level rises to a higher level. So, they are as well a timely remedy to fighting stress "arrows" in an early stage of the attack. Apart from this, massage chairs should also remind you to take pauses of relaxation regularly.

CHAPTER 7:
HOW DO YOU TELL THE DIFFERENCE BETWEEN BACK PAIN AND KIDNEY INFECTION PAIN?

As back pain seems to be a part of our lives, which can affect anybody at any time it is crucial to find out what type of back pain is involved. Back pain might occur periodically, stay for a brief time, and then quickly disappear. In this case, this kind of pain is to be considered acute back pain. That kind of pain could be taken care of with medication and rest.

However, if the pain remains for more than three months, this pain is to be regarded as chronic back pain. So, the pain duration determines its categorization. This is also true for those who are suffering from kidney infections since kidney infections also come in two different forms: chronic (long duration of gradual pain) and acute (short duration but strong pain).

Mostly, kidney infections will cause pain. This pain may resemble lower-back discomfort. The kidneys are situated on either side of the spinal column just above the hip. Your kidneys are two organs that lie within the back abdominal cavity of the torso. The kidneys' function is to make sure that proper water and electrolyte are in balance. Moreover, it accounts for the regulation of the blood and any waste that should be excreted through the urine. If the same area of your back is in pain, kidney pain and back pain will often be subject to be confused with one another. However, if you are experiencing back pain near the kidney area, you should immediately consult a doctor.

If you are suffering from a kidney infection, the discomfort will originate within the kidney and radiate towards the lower back. This is recognized as referred pain. That is the reason why extremely often kidney infection is confused with low-back pain. So how do you tell the difference between back pain and kidney infection pain?

First, as your kidneys are in the lower half of your abdomen, near your back, pain that radiates around the kidneys is often sensed to be in the lower sections of the back. This, of course, can lead to confusion if this is an area that is regularly subject to strain in your daily activities. But if you are suffering from pain in the upper area of your back, up to the shoulder area, that pain area will provide more evidence that your discomfort is not due to a kidney infection. In this case, you are much more likely to experience back pain.

Second, if you are facing a kidney infection, then the pain that is radiating from the kidney will be sharp and harsh. In this case, heat and massage therapy will fail to relieve the pain that comes in waves. Typical back pain can be relieved with massage and a heating pad application. By the way, this is a great method to tell if you are experiencing kidney problems or just some discomfort in your back. We have already discussed the benefits of massage therapy in the last chapter. So, before you consult a physician you can take this simple test by applying massage therapy. If the pain still prevails, you should seek the professional opinion of a physician.

Often, kidney pain is due to kidney stones and kidney infections. The symptoms of kidney infection or kidney stones could involve pain throughout urination, blood within the urine, or fever with accompanying chills. It is quite simple for your doctor to find out if you are affected by either of these cases. Your physician will just need to press on the kidneys at the time of physical examination. If there is a shooting pain within this region, you can be quite sure you are suffering from a kidney infection or kidney stones.

Kidney stones are severe. Sometimes, the pain caused by them is compared to the pain from childbirth. As for kidney infection, the pain is rather sharp and flanking with sensitivity to the touch.

Third, to check the level of the white blood cells in your body doctors will most likely ask you for a urine sample. The result of this sample gives valuable clues to whether your body is fighting an infection or not.

Unfortunately, kidney pain could also be due to much more severe reasons that might involve kidney cancer, polycystic kidney disease, blocked urine flow, and bladder spasms. But as a rule, the symptoms of a quite ordinary kidney infection come on rapidly and vanish once the course of medication is over. Moreover, if you happen to suffer from a kidney infection, the pain will happen on one side of the back, above the waist but just below the rib cage. Besides, the pain might be more intense as the bladder gets full, or it may even hit you towards the genital area. As already mentioned, during this time you might have bouts of vomiting, pain while urination, blood within the urine as well as fever. To put it bluntly: if your pain is happening with the blood in the urine (not always visible), burning during urination, nausea, and fever, you can be sure that you are suffering from a kidney infection. So, after the diagnosis is confirmed how is kidney infection to be treated?

As kidney infections are caused by bacteria that get into the bladder and move to the kidneys, taking antibiotics is the usual form of treatment for a kidney infection. If you wait and do not receive treatment for a kidney infection, you might end up damaging your kidneys. So, make sure if you think you may have a kidney infection to see your doctor right away and get the proper treatment.

If your case is to be considered severe, your doctor will probably give you a shot of antibiotics. Moreover, you may get pain medication and anti-nausea medicine on prescription that will fight these symptoms. The tension in the lower back will fade gradually as the infection goes away.

So, after we discussed the symptoms of a kidney infection, how is back pain to be distinguished from kidney infection pain? Many different things cause back pain in the lower half of the back. If you experience trouble from twisting, bending, or even sitting, tense muscles are the common cause. But these symptoms could also point to a damaged herniated disk. When stiff and sore joints coincide with a stiff and sore lower back this will more likely account for arthritis that is either in a fledgling or flaring stage. You can get low-back pain from some very simple things like walking in high heels or maybe stretching improperly. If you are suffering from a kidney infection, this too can develop into low-back pains and become very painful. In case you are expecting you should be aware that pregnancy is commonly responsible for lower pressure in the back, as the ligaments in the abdomen need to stretch for childbirth. In the next chapter, we will take a closer look at how much back pain is normal after pregnancy before getting concerned.

Suffering from severe pain of any part of the back can also be resulting from a spinal fracture, which is a very serious issue. In this case, most likely you will need to go to the emergency room as soon as possible. If, however, your muscles are stretched, torn, or twisted, the pain will probably be centered around this particular region. The pain may ignite either in the lower back, radiating in between shoulder blades, and moving below the waist or over the spinal column. This kind of pain will worsen with the increase of movement and fade away while resting. If you should experience this kind of interdependency, you will be most likely not suffering from a kidney infection.

Now, knowing this, if you are suffering from low-back pain after you pulled a muscle, herniated a spinal disc, or strained your back, then you will have the answer for the pain: it will not be from a kidney infection.

So, after you have the answer for the pain's source, how is back pain to be treated? First of all, you need to know that if you suffer from low-back pain, this pain will not as easily be remedied as the pain from a kidney infection. Using antibiotics or even shots of antibiotics will not be the answer to your pain issue as your pain source is not due to an amassment of bacteria.

Low-back pain can be treated by: Heating pads, physical therapy, and oral pain medication. In those cases, in which pain is a result of herniated discs, strains, overdoing exercise, improper stretching, and back spasms, there will be a more extensive treatment necessary. For further and much more detailed back pain treatment methods, please check chapter five ("what are the best methods to relieve back pain?"). By now, you know low-back pain triggered by these events is much more different from low-back pain that is due to a kidney infection.

So, let us sum up these differences one more time:

1) Kidney pain and back pain can often and easily be confused with one another. To be sure about the rights diagnosis you should visit your physician.

2) The pain in the lower part of the back can be a result of pulled muscles, herniated disks, arthritis, pregnancy, or fracture of the spine. Kidney pain can also be due to kidney stones, kidney infection, kidney cancer, and polycystic kidney disease.

3) Back pain can be cured with a heat compress and massage. Kidney pain will not be relieved using these methods.

CHAPTER 8:
HOW MUCH BACK PAIN IS NORMAL AFTER PREGNANCY BEFORE GETTING CONCERNED?

In the previous chapter, it has already been mentioned that expecting women should consider that pregnancy is commonly responsible for lower pressure in the back as the ligaments in the abdomen need to stretch for childbirth. So, back pain during pregnancy should not take you by surprise. However, it still deserves attention and alertness. Actually, without exception expecting women will have to undergo some kind of back pain during their pregnancy. Moreover, during pregnancy expecting, women continue to complain about increasing back pain. This is due to several reasons:

1) Expecting women tend to gain weight. At the beginning of pregnancy, this may be a more or less subtle process. But as childbirth is in sight gaining weight speeds up and becomes more and more obvious.

2) Expecting women tend to take a completely new road as their hormones are pursuing a quite different goal since the beginning of pregnancy, which is relaxing the muscles and ligaments throughout your body to make them elastic for the day of childbirth. But the good news is you do not need to be hopelessly committed to the painful impact of this ongoing process. Many times, you can counteract or even prevent back pain during pregnancy. Let us take a look at seven ways to hold back pain during pregnancy at bay:

1. Keep a good posture

As your baby grows, you will be more and more inclined to slouch as your center of gravity is shifting constantly forward. To balance this process of bending forward many expecting women take quite opposite steps by leaning back excessively. This, as a result, can put tension on the muscles in your lower back and contribute to back pain during pregnancy. Given this, keep a good posture by applying these principles:

-Stand up straight and tall. Stand on tiptoes every once in a while.

-Hold your chest high while catching your breath.

-Keep your shoulders back and stress-relieved.

-Do not lock your knees.

If you need to stand for an extended time, make sure to put one foot on a low step stool for a rest. Take time to pause frequently. Keeping a good posture implies not only your way of standing but also the way you use to sit. Choose a chair that enhances your efforts to keep your upper back and neck constantly straight. Place a pregnancy pillow behind your lower back. For further relaxation, consider propping your feet on a low stool.

2. Mind the right equipment

As we have already discussed in the previous chapter, you can get low-back pain from some very simple things like walking in high heels. In particular, expecting women will need to avoid this mistake. So, wearing low-heeled shoes with good arch support should be a priority during pregnancy. Moreover, wearing maternity pants with a low waistband could also be of supportive value. You might also take into consideration wearing a maternity support belt. As for maternity support belts, their effectiveness is contentious. Some women seem to benefit from them; others cannot even tell if they make any major difference.

3. Lift in a proper manner

Whenever you need to lift an object, you will have to make sure to squat down before lifting. The lifting power must come from your legs. Despite the object's weight, make it a habit to squat down. Never bend down at the waist or lift with your back. Do not feel shy or uncomfortable asking for support if you need it.

4. Sleep on your side

To release your back from undue tension, you should spend most of your night sleeping on your side rather than on your back. Make it a habit to keep one or even both knees bent. You might place one pillow between your knees and another under your abdomen, or use a full-length body pillow.

5. Use heat or massage

Heating pads can make a great contribution to heat your back and thus relieve the tension. Rubbing your back involves tense-relieving qualities, too. A professional prenatal massage might be the best and most rewarding method to relieve and even prevent back pain if applied regularly.

6. Make physical activity your daily routine

If you make it your priority to pursue physical activity regularly, you will keep your back strong. As a consequence, you will relieve back pain during pregnancy. However, always consider gentle activities such as walking or swimming. You should also consider doing the following highly recommendable exercise:

Cat Stretch: Stretch your lower back. Rest on your hands and knees with your head in line with your back. Pull in your stomach, rounding your back slightly. Hold for several seconds, and then relax your stomach and back keeping your back as flat as possible. See the exercise demonstration below:

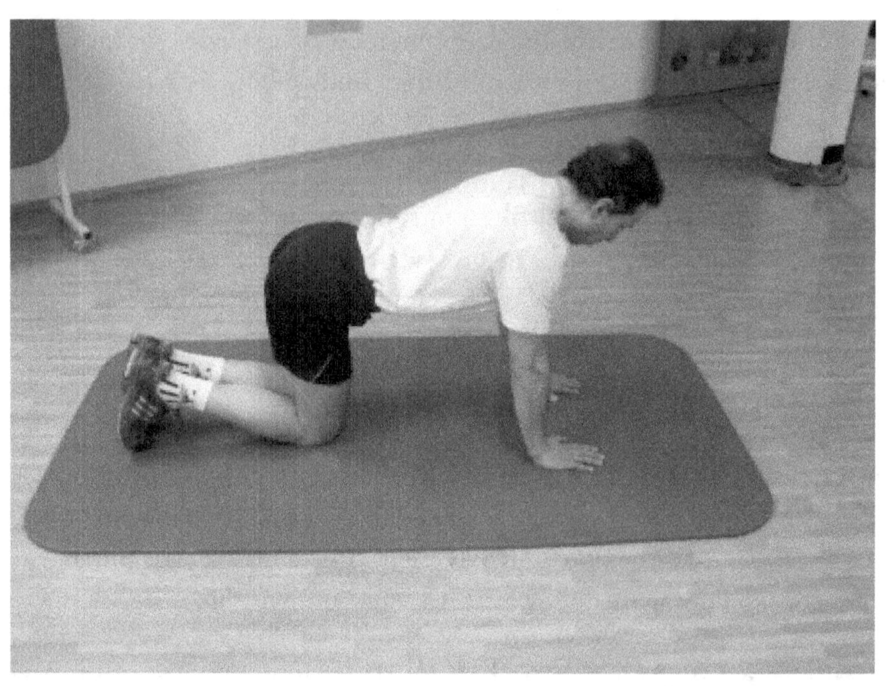

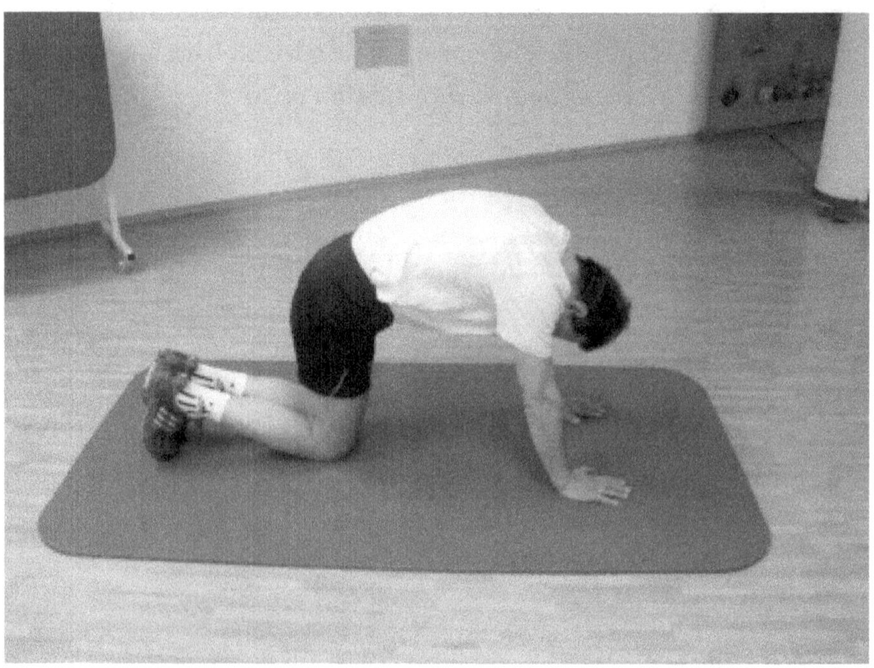

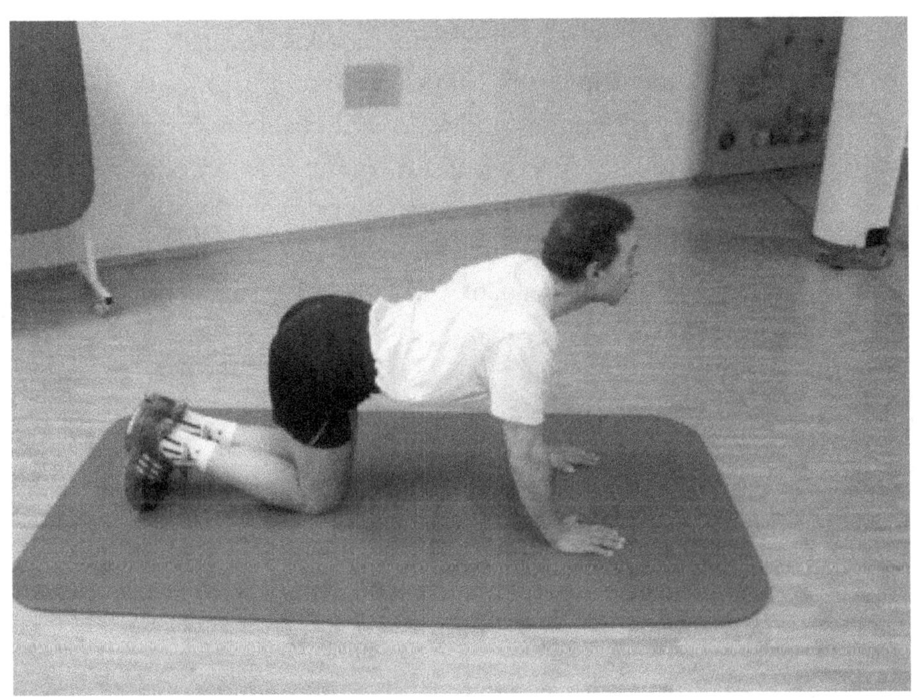

7. Apply complementary therapies

To battle back pain, some expecting women experience tremendous relief from back pain during pregnancy by applying acupuncture. Chiropractic treatment seems to provide beneficial pain-easing effects for some women, too. If you are considering a complementary therapy such as these, please consult your physician first to obtain his opinion on it. Because your physician should confirm that your back pain is due to your condition of pregnancy before considering these complementary therapy methods.

So, is back pain during pregnancy quite normal? Or how much pain are expecting women supposed to take before getting concerned?

Summing up: as already mentioned at the beginning of this chapter, common back pain during pregnancy might be normal but should not be treated lightly. If you should not experience any relief from the self-care strategies described above, you should consult your physician. Medication such as acetaminophen (Tylenol, others) is not always a disputable matter. However, before jumping into this, consult your physician first.

Besides, you need to be aware that pertinacious backache might be signaling preterm labor. Severe and lasting back pain or back pain in combination with vaginal bleeding or discharge could indicate an underlying problem that needs immediate remedial measure. As a result, whenever the self-care strategies discussed above fail to provide you genuine relief from your back pain or your back pain is accompanied by much more serious symptoms as mentioned, your back pain is NOT normal during pregnancy. Thus, you need to be concerned and consult your physician as soon as possible.

CHAPTER 9:
HOW IS SCIATICA PAIN DIFFERENT FROM BACK PAIN?

If your lower back has been aching for an extended time, an acute attack of sciatic pain, or sciatica, might be the source. Whenever muscle tissue, bone, or an intervertebral disc pressures the nerve root of the sciatic nerve, sciatic pain ignites. As a consequence, nerve roots that are linked to sciatic nerves turn out to be pinched and inflamed, which makes this condition very painful.

Sciatica produces sudden, traveling pain that usually begins in the lower back and radiates down through the legs. This sort of back pain can be chronic, acute, or sub-acute. As already discussed in chapter one, low-back pain is also manifested in these three types of pain.

So, when is back pain to be considered acute? When your back pain lasts for just a few hours or days, your pain is to be regarded as acute. If the pain should cover at least three months, then your backache is considered to be sub-acute. In case, you do not experience any relief from back pain for longer than three months, your back pain has become a chronic issue.

So, how is sciatic pain to be distinguished from back pain? First, sciatica pain differs from "normal" back pain as it impacts three areas of the body in a downward direction. As a rule, sciatic pain starts in the lower back, moves to the gluteus maximum muscles, and ends up in the leg muscles. Second, sciatic pain has three phases. In the first phase, you face a sudden manifestation of the pain coming out of the blue. In the second phase, the pain arrives at its peak before it starts to ease down in the third phase.

Very often, the three areas that are involved induce numbness, tingling, or weakness.

But there are also different symptoms sciatica sufferers do complain about. Some may notice burning or tingling pain on only one side of their buttock or in only one leg that becomes worse once they sit down. As the sciatic nerve runs down each leg it diverges into two segments at the tailbone. That is why some may experience different symptoms on each side of the body. However, as symptoms become very intense in the second phase some people might even have a hard time standing up or walk.

Although the symptoms of back pain are different from sciatic pain, sciatica is also due to an underlying problem of the lower back. Spinal stenosis or a herniated disc could be responsible for the excessive nerve compression or nerve irritation. To treat sciatica properly, it is crucial to make out the reason or the source of the pain. Pain-relieving drugs should only be prescribed until the source of pain is made out. The cause of sciatic pain is decisive for the type of treatment you need to consider. Treatment may include pain medication, exercise, physical therapy, or even surgery if necessary.

So, what are the common causes for sciatica?

Common sciatic pain is due to the following five back problems:

1. Piriformis syndrome:

This occurs once the sciatic nerve is irritated if it crosses the piriformis muscle behind. In case the piriformis muscle pinches or even aggravates nerve roots that contain the sciatic nerve, you will suffer from sciatic pain.

2. Sacroiliac joint dysfunction:

This issue is due to an irritation in the sacroiliac joint, which is located near the bottom of your spine. This may also trigger discomfort in L5 nerves, which are next to the peak of your sacroiliac joint, leading to sciatic pain.

3. Lumbar herniated disc:

Herniated discs result from leaking out of soft inner cores of discs known as nucleus pulposus. It irritates the adjacent nervous roots as it leaves the spine.

4. Degenerative disc disease:

Disc degeneration is to be considered a completely ordinary process that is often observed in elderly people.

5. Lumbar spinal stenosis:

This is a condition that generally causes sciatica because of the narrowing spinal canal. Particularly, people at the age of sixty and more are affected by this kind of sciatic pain.

Sciatica might also be the result of an injury or event. Suffering people are often between the ages of thirty and fifty.

Sciatic pain appears to be due to a lingering process triggered by general everyday wear and tear on the lower spine. The clinical diagnosis of sciatica is referred to as "radiculopathy." This simply means that a disc within the spine has protruded from its normal position in the vertebral column. Because of this, it is putting pressure on the nerve root (radicular nerve) in the lower back, which forms part of the sciatic nerve.

So, after discussing the sciatic causes, how can sciatic pain be relieved? Let us take a look at the following sciatic exercises:

1) In most cases, exercising regularly has a pain-relieving impact it strengthens muscles within the back and legs. Taking a walk is one of the easiest ways to exercise these muscles. So, make regular walking a habit. Walking up to three miles a day at a brisk pace will certainly have a fantastic pain-relieving impact. It is a great way to strengthen your lower back. Besides, it is considered to be a low-impact exercise that enhances the strength and flexibility of your muscles, which ultimately relieves sciatic pain.

2) Aerobic exercise works great in the same way and with the same benefits. It strengthens muscles associated with sciatic pain. In general, aerobic is an awesome method to achieve entire body fitness.

3) To set the records straight, working out regularly always outdoes bed rest and is thus much more recommended to ease sciatic pain. As the cause of sciatic pain is decisive for the type of treatment you need to consider the fitness program is to be tailored to the underlying cause of pain. Any personalized workout program intended to relieve sciatic pain should involve:

a) Proper Workout: if you do the right exercises the wrong way, these exercises might not only appear to be completely useless, but they could even aggravate your pain issue.

b) Specific Analysis: any medical workout program has to aim at finding out the pain source behind the discomfort in the patient's sciatica treatment.

c) Core strengthening of muscles: sciatica workouts should primarily focus on the strengthening of back muscles and the abdomen. Thus, it stabilizes your spine making you much less susceptible to sciatic pain.

d) Avoid specific exercises: currently, you might face many sciatic exercises promising to relieve pain. However, there are some exercises that you should not include in your program. As a basic rule, any exercise that puts pressure on the lower back is to be avoided. In particular, you should avoid the following exercises:

1) Exercising the abdomen is a good way to strengthen your spine. However, avoid sit-ups with both legs straight because in this position excessive pressure is put on the spinal discs.

2) Some of the most dangerous backbone exercises are deadlifts leading to spine pain and severe aggravation of sciatic pain. Unfortunately, a lot of young men brag about their weight lifting achievements but are blind to the long-term devastating effects of lifting these heavyweights.

3) Always avoid having barbells upon your shoulders while squatting. This exercise might have a hazardous impact on your lower spine. As the entire pressure of the barbell is resting on the spine, this exercise can induce an overall compression of the spine and intervertebral discs which is the cause of herniation and pinched nerves. As already mentioned, the pain caused by herniated discs radiates toward the buttocks and legs.

4) Any kind of exercise that heavily stretches your hamstring muscle is to be avoided in any case. Because any stretching that affects the hamstring also pulls the root of the sciatic nerve. This, however, can do more harm than good.

Summing up: you should make proper exercises part of your daily routine and not just a petty evil that you schedule whenever it fits your daily program. So, with sufficient care as well as the discipline you will experience dramatic relief from your sciatic pain.

If you want to learn awesome sciatic exercises, you should watch the video series of **Esther Ekhart** (https://for-ever-fit.net/yoga-exercises).

CHAPTER 10:
WHAT IS THE BEST BED FOR BACK PAIN RELIEF?

Many people wonder whether there are beds that have a beneficial impact on back and spine health. There are these beds. However, it is more rather the mattress that qualifies the bed than the bed itself. Given this, a foam mattress is highly recommendable for those people who may suffer from back pain issues. Moreover, people who are suffering from insomnia and thus are desperately looking for a comfortable night's sleep, should not avoid the investment into a foam mattress. Insomnia might be due to several other reasons than resulting from an improper mattress. But often, sleeping disorders can be traced back to simple causes like having the "wrong bed." Unfortunately, many people seem to be careless when it comes to investing time and money to choose the right mattress. As a consequence, they may experience severe back problems and other issues in the long run. As a result, this might push people to take radical steps to make sure they have a goodnight's sleep such as sleep-inducing drugs and sedatives.

As in chapter one already discussed, eighty percent of Americans complain of low-back pain at some point in their lives. We also pointed out that these causes might have an acute, sub-acute, or chronic quality. Fortunately, the easiest way to treat back pain occurs during sleep. As back pain can get worse by simply sleeping in the wrong position, it can also be often relieved by just using the proper mattress support. So, before we can value the benefits of a foam mattress, we should take a closer look at the standard spring mattress.

So, what are spring mattresses all about? Springs are often associated with their ability to push back against the body and thus provide support. However, the issue is that this pushing-back process is always delivered with equal force. As human body parts use to differ in their weight (some are heavier and others are lighter), spring mattresses do not take this different weight distribution into account. As a result, as spring mattresses always use to push back with the same force, they will necessarily support different parts of the body with the same power.

This might not sound alarming in the first place. But as a matter of fact, the human body is created to have different pressure points of which some require much more intense support than others when we sleep. The lower back is one of these pressure points that are subject to more support. Because, first, the lower back is where most of us carry most of our weight, and second, it combines a sophisticated network of nerves, discs, and bones, which makes it one of the most sensitive areas of the body.

Considering this, studies showed that spring mattresses will necessarily fail when it comes to offering different body parts different support. This might be a reason for jactitation (extreme restlessness and tossing in bed), poor blood circulation, and a lousy night's sleep. Using poor mattress support could even result in symptoms like insomnia, aches, pains, and aggravation of existing injuries. So, people who suffer from acute, sub-acute or particularly chronic back pain should forgo spring mattresses.

Now, let us review the benefits of a foam mattress. Before foam mattresses became public in the early nineties they were used in hospitals for patients who were confined to bed for quite a time. As spring mattresses were used by default in earlier days, these patients were forced to spend weeks or even months lying in bed on a spring mattress. As a result, they started complaining about painful sores, even gangrene, due to poor blood circulation. But most surprisingly, this was not the case with foam mattresses. Shortly after this, foam mattresses were offered to the public.

So, what makes the use of foam so outstanding? To put it simply, the foam takes into consideration that different body parts require unequal treatment due to their differing weight. In contrast to spring mattresses, foam molds to a person's body and provides body parts with the proper support they need. As a result, these mattresses make sure to provide an even bodyweight distribution. That is exactly what spring mattresses fail to achieve. Studies showed that people who sleep on foam mattresses suffer much less from jactitation and therefore enjoy a goodnight's sleep. Moreover, even as for the duration these mattresses outdo spring mattresses by far. They will support a person's body weight for decades without fail.

Is there any downside when it comes to using foam mattresses? The nature of foam accounts for its susceptibility to temperature. This simply means that the room's temperature determines how fast foam can deploy its molding qualities. For instance, if you use to sleep in a cold room, the longer it will take the foam to adjust to your body weight. At worst, foam mattresses can become hard as a rock if you have the habit to leave the windows open even on a stone-cold winter night. However, this sleeping habit might rather be considered exceptional. So, that is the downside but one that can be avoided. The only type of memory foam that is not sensitive to temperature is called "essential natural memory foam". The foam is sensitive to temperature warm temperature makes foam displaying its molding characteristics at a much more accelerated pace. So, during the summer months, these mattresses will mold to your body in a matter of seconds providing your body parts with the proper support they need.

Summing up: foam mattresses should be your first and only choice if you have been suffering from back pain after sleeping or due to the reasons mentioned above. In addition to the recommendations such as exercise, proper posture, and the many others discussed, foam mattresses offer a great service when it comes to relieving your back pain permanently.

Notes:

45

<u>**Notes:**</u>

46

Don't miss out!

Visit the website below and you can sign up to receive emails whenever Dr. Robertino Bedenian publishes a new book. There's no charge and no obligation.

https://books2read.com/r/B-A-YQGQ-AABSB

BOOKS 2 READ

Connecting independent readers to independent writers.

Also by Dr. Robertino Bedenian

Fitness Over 60 For Women – How to Stay Fit And Healthy As You Age
Does Back Pain Go Away? 10 Answers To The Most Acute Back Pain Issues
Massage Bible - A Beginners Guide To Western And Eastern Massage Therapy
Going Vegan - How To Vegan Without Going Crazy
Chiropraktik - Was Steckt Eigentlich Dahinter?
Massagen: Ein Überblick Über Westliche Und Östliche Massagetechniken
Natuerlich Abnehmen, Schlank Und Endlich Fit Sein
P.S. Ich Liebe Dich: Wenn Liebe So Einfach Wäre
Was Tun Bei Rückenschmerzen, Bandscheibenvorfall Und Ischiasschmerzen: 10
Antworten Zu Den Häufigsten Fragen Bei Rückenschmerzen
Was Tun Gegen Schlafapnoe, Schlafstörungen Und Schnarchen
Self-Help Books for Women – How to Overcome Depression, Anxiety,
Divorce, Addiction, and Trauma
Your Super Gut Feeling Restored – How to Restore Your Life Energy and
Overall Health from The Inside Out

Watch for more at https://booksummarypublishing.com.

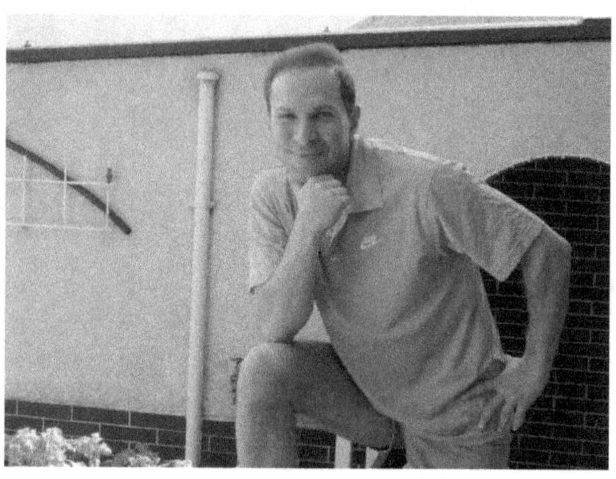

About the Author

Dr. Robertino Bedenian is a qualified fitness instructor accredited by the German Olympic Committee, a health and nutrition expert, and the author of several books on diet, health, and fitness!

For more than twenty years he has been a fitness coach at the sports university teaching aerobics, back gymnastics, stretching, high-intensity interval training (HIIT), power gymnastics, and athletic sports.

On his website, he has published more than 300 articles about the vegan lifestyle covering diet and health recommendations, detoxication programs,

fitness guidelines, and disease-related topics. He is part of a family with an orthopedic surgeon, a physical therapist, an osteopath, and an alternative practitioner.

He is also the founder of the brand "**Going Vegan**" selling high-quality supplements for optimal health.

You are more than welcome to check his website for more details: https://goingveganhealthbenefits.com.

His brand has been awarded continuously with 5-star feedback by customers for its outstanding product quality.

Dr. Bedenian is also the founder of the book company "**Book Summary Publishing**" publishing summaries and workbooks of Amazon #1 bestselling non-fiction books.

If you want to learn more about the summaries and workbooks that he has published so far, please visit his website: